Eat Well, Live Well

"A Guide to Nutrition and Energy for Busy People"

By

Dwight W. Gagne

DISCLAIMER

Contents

Introduction

The cornerstone of health and well-being is proper nutrition. The foods and beverages that we consume have an impact on every facet of our lives, from our physical performance and mental clarity to our spirits and the amount of energy that we have. In today's fast-paced and hectic world, however, it can be challenging to find the time and the drive to maintain a healthy diet and drink plenty of water. I prepared this book to assist you in making sensible and uncomplicated decisions that will provide nourishment to both your body and your mind without causing you to go bankrupt or take up an excessive amount of your valuable time. In this book, you will discover the basics of nutrition, such as the roles and functions of macronutrients (carbohydrates, proteins, and fats) and micronutrients (vitamins and minerals). You will also discover how to combine your hectic schedule with nutrition, with practical recommendations on meal planning, quick and healthy snack ideas, and the significance of water. You will also find out how to choose foods that will boost your energy and keep you going throughout the day, as well as how to optimize your nutrition for exercise and recovery. Whether you are a beginner or a nutrition expert, this book will provide you with the knowledge and tools you need to improve your health and wellness. By following the suggestions and recipes in this book, you will not only feel better but also look better, perform better, and live better. So, what are you waiting for? Let's get started!

Chapter One

Understanding Macronutrients

Your body needs a lot of macronutrients to perform at its best. They consist of fat, protein, and carbs. Your body gets its energy, structure, and activities from them.

Your body uses carbohydrates as its primary energy source, particularly for your muscles and brain. They consist of simple sugar molecules, such as disaccharides and monosaccharides, or complex sugar molecules, known as polysaccharides. Whole grains, fruits, vegetables, beans, and legumes are good sources of complex carbohydrates. They are abundant in antioxidants, vitamins, minerals, and fiber. Processed meals, sweets, and refined grains all include simple carbohydrates. They are rapidly absorbed and digested, which raises insulin and blood sugar levels.

 Because it is composed of the amino acids that give your cells, tissues, and organs their structure and functionality, protein is the building block of your body. Protein is necessary for immune system function, growth, repair, hormone synthesis, and enzyme activity. Plants (beans, legumes, nuts, seeds, and soy products) and animals (meat, eggs, dairy, and fish) are the two main sources of protein. Plant sources might not include all the necessary amino acids your body needs, while animal sources have all of them. To ensure that you are getting all the amino acids you require, it is crucial to consume a range of plant-based proteins.

With 9 calories per gram of fat compared to 4 calories per gram of carbohydrates and protein, fat is the most concentrated source of energy for your body. In addition, fat is necessary for hormone synthesis, neuron transmission, brain development, and the absorption of fat-soluble vitamins (A, D, E, and K). Saturated, unsaturated, and trans fats are the three categories of fat. At room temperature, saturated fats remain solid and are present in animal products like cheese, butter, and fatty meats, as well as certain plant oils like coconut and palm oil. Nuts, seeds, avocados, fatty fish, and plant oils (including olive, canola, and sunflower oil) are sources of unsaturated fats, which are liquid at room temperature. Trans fats are produced artificially in processed foods (baked products, fried foods, and margarine) by adding hydrogen to vegetable oils. Because they can reduce your risk of heart disease and stroke, unsaturated fats are typically better for you than saturated and trans fats.

 The following ranges are advised for the consumption of macronutrients:

 Carbs make up 45–65% of all calories.

10–35% of total calories come from protein.

20–35% of calories come from fat.

These ranges, however, could change based on your age, sex, degree of activity, desired level of health, and individual preferences. The benefits of varying macronutrient intakes for different individuals may vary based on their unique demands and circumstances. For instance, those with diabetes may need to restrict their intake of carbohydrates, but frequent exercisers may require a higher protein intake to maintain their muscles.

You can utilize online calculators, applications, or formulas that estimate your calorie and macronutrient requirements based on your goals and personal information to determine your macronutrient needs. Additionally, you can use meal diaries, apps, or websites to keep track of your macronutrient ratios and food intake. These techniques, however, may not take into consideration other elements that impact your nutrition, such as food quality, portion sizes, nutritional density, and bioavailability. They are also not always precise or dependable. As a result, it is wise to speak with a qualified dietitian or nutritionist who can offer you individualized, fact-based advice regarding the amount and requirements of macronutrients.

1. Carbohydrates

Basic biomolecules, such as carbohydrates, are essential to the operation of all living things. These substances, which are mostly made up of carbon, hydrogen, and oxygen, provide energy for several different biological functions. Understanding the role of carbohydrates is crucial to appreciate their influence on human health, metabolism, and general welfare.

Three basic forms of carbohydrates can be distinguished: monosaccharides, disaccharides, and polysaccharides. The most basic types of carbohydrates are called monosaccharides, and they include glucose and fructose. These molecules are the building blocks of more complicated structures. Disaccharides are composed of two monosaccharide units joined together, such as lactose and sucrose. Large molecules called polysaccharides, which include cellulose and starch, are created when monosaccharide units are repeated.

Energy production for biological processes is one of the main uses of carbohydrates. One monosaccharide that is particularly significant in this context is glucose. Cells obtain energy from glucose molecules through a sequence of metabolic activities, including glycolysis and cellular respiration. After that, this energy is used for a variety of physiological processes, such as the synthesis of vital biomolecules and the contraction of muscles.

Additionally, carbohydrates are essential for the storage of energy. In humans, extra glucose is metabolized into glycogen, which is then stored in the muscles and liver. The breakdown of glycogen releases glucose when the body needs more energy. This dynamic control over glucose levels contributes to a continuous supply of energy for biological processes.

Carbohydrates have roles in energy production, but they are also essential for cellular communication. Glycolipids and glycoproteins, which are carbohydrates found on the cell surface, play a role in signaling and cell recognition. These molecules demonstrate the variety of roles that carbohydrates play in biological systems by being essential for immunological responses, fertilization, and tissue formation.

Dietary carbohydrates play a major role in the nutrition of humans. Carbohydrate-rich foods include fruits, vegetables, grains, and legumes. Carbohydrates are categorized as simple or complex based on the structure of their molecules and how quickly they break down during digestion. Blood glucose levels rise quickly due to the quick absorption of simple carbohydrates, also known as sugars. Complex carbs, on the other hand, which are present in foods like whole grains and vegetables, digest more slowly and release energy gradually.

Research and debate over the health effects of carbs are still ongoing. Diets high in carbohydrates have been connected to diseases including type 2 diabetes and obesity, highlighting the need to know the kind and amount of carbohydrates consumed. The glycemic index, which assigns a number to carbohydrates according to how they affect blood sugar, has grown to be an important tool for those trying to control their blood sugar levels when making dietary decisions.

It is important to remember that not all carbohydrates are created equal. In general, whole, unprocessed foods are seen to be healthier sources of carbs than processed, high-sugar diets. Plant-based meals contain fiber, a form of carbohydrate that is essential for digestive health and has been linked to a lower risk of chronic illnesses.

Carbohydrates and controlling weight have a complicated and intricate relationship. Even though various low-carb diets have become more popular for helping people lose weight, research is still being done on the sustainability and long-term implications of these strategies. A balanced diet that includes enough amounts of fats, proteins, and carbohydrates is essential for overall health.

Not only are carbohydrates essential to human nutrition but they are also found in the diets of other living things. Carbohydrates generated by photosynthesis give plants energy for expansion and growth. Carbohydrates are derived from plant-based meals for herbivores, but they are ingested by carnivores indirectly. The complex network of nutrient transport illustrated by this illustrates how interrelated ecosystems are.

Carbohydrate research is useful in many different industries and goes beyond nutrition and biology. For example, the fermentation of carbohydrates is a common step in the generation of biofuels. Carbohydrates are also essential to the food business since they contribute to texture, flavor, and preservation. Optimizing these processes requires a thorough understanding of the chemical and physical characteristics of carbohydrates.

 Because they are a fundamental source of energy, a structural element, and a signaling molecule in living things, carbohydrates are essential to life. Their many roles highlight how crucial it is to include a sensible and balanced approach to the consumption of carbohydrates in the diet as well as in larger biological processes. The complexities of glucose metabolism and their effects on health are still being uncovered by the ongoing study, which also provides fresh perspectives on the dynamic interactions between these vital biomolecules and the complex web of life.

2. Proteins

Proteins are necessary macromolecules that are vital to the structure and operation of all living things. These complex molecules, which consist of chains of amino acids, have a role in a multitude of biological activities, ranging from enzyme catalysis to cellular structure. Since proteins are the building blocks of life and perform a variety of tasks inside cells, they are extremely important in the biological domain.

The amino acid sequence forms the basis of protein structure. Twenty distinct amino acids can be combined in different ways to generate a large variety of proteins. The function of a protein is dictated by its three-dimensional structure, which is determined by its specific amino acid sequence. One of the main features of proteins is the intricate link that exists between structure and function.

The four main structural levels of proteins are quaternary, tertiary, secondary, and primary. The linear arrangement of amino acids in a polypeptide chain is referred to as the fundamental structure. This sequence is an essential component of genetic information since genes encode it. Alpha helices and beta sheets are formed as a result of interactions like hydrogen bonding, which give rise to the secondary structure. A single polypeptide chain folds in three dimensions to generate tertiary structure, whereas numerous polypeptide chains interact to form functional protein complexes in quaternary structure.

The functions of proteins are very diverse. A class of proteins called enzymes facilitates and speeds up biological reactions by acting as catalysts. Another protein that is essential for carrying oxygen in the blood is hemoglobin. Another class of proteins that are vital to the immune system's function of protecting the body from infections are antibodies.

Cell structure and function are entirely dependent on proteins. Tissues, including skin, tendons, and bones, are supported and strengthened by structural proteins like collagen. Movement is made possible by the muscles' contracting proteins, myosin and actin. Transport proteins help molecules travel through biological barriers. Examples of these proteins are present in cell membranes.

Translation is the process that creates new proteins, a process known as protein biosynthesis. This complex process results in the translation of the information contained in messenger RNA (mRNA) into a particular amino acid sequence, which in turn forms a functioning protein. The cellular machinery called ribosomes is in charge of synthesizing proteins. It reads the mRNA code and assembles amino acids according to genetic instructions.

Protein synthesis regulation is a strictly regulated process. Certain proteins can be produced at different rates by cells in response to internal or external stimuli. This regulation helps maintain the organism's general homeostasis by ensuring that the cellular machinery generates the appropriate proteins at the appropriate times.

The folding of proteins is essential to function. Misfolded proteins, which are linked to a number of illnesses, including neurodegenerative conditions like Alzheimer's and Parkinson's, can result from improper folding. Chaperone proteins help other proteins fold correctly, avoiding misfolding and preserving cellular integrity.

Dietary proteins are necessary for an organism's nourishment. When proteins from food are digested in humans, they are converted into amino acids and then taken up by the blood. The body uses these amino acids as the building blocks to synthesize new proteins. Because the body is unable to produce essential amino acids, eating is the only way to get them.

Post-translational modifications, or changes to the amino acid sequence following translation, can occur in proteins. These alterations may have an impact on the location, activity, and stability of proteins within the cell. Phosphorylation, glycosylation, and acetylation are a few types of post-translational modifications.

Technological developments in biotechnology have made it possible to produce recombinant proteins. Through the use of genetic engineering techniques, particular genes can be inserted into host species to produce desired proteins for use in industry, medicine, or study. This has completely changed industries like medicine, where recombinant proteins are used as diagnostic and therapeutic tools.

Because they function as the molecular machinery that powers the various operations inside cells, proteins are essential to life. Proteins are essential for the proper operation and integrity of living things, providing anything from structural support to biochemical reaction catalysis. Comprehending the complexities of protein synthesis, structure, and function has broad ramifications spanning domains including nutrition, biotechnology, and medicine. There is still a great deal of room for ground-breaking discoveries and advances across a wide range of scientific fields as study into the intricacies of proteins continues.

3. Fats

Given their many vital roles in the body, fats play a significant role in our diet. They are one of the three macronutrients that, along with proteins and carbs, provide energy and are essential for preserving general health. Even though fats are frequently misinterpreted and vilified, it is critical to acknowledge their significance and the necessity of consuming them in moderation.

Saturated, unsaturated, and trans fats are the three main categories of dietary fats. When ingested in excess, saturated fats—which are frequently found in animal products like meat and dairy—have been linked to an elevated risk of heart disease. Conversely, unsaturated fats, found in foods like seeds, nuts, and vegetable oils, are thought to be heart-healthy and good for general health.

Energy production is one of the fats' main purposes. Compared to proteins and carbs, fats provide more calories per gram, making them a concentrated source of energy for the body. The body uses stored fats to provide energy when it requires more than what is readily available from carbohydrates. This procedure is particularly important when fasting or consuming fewer carbohydrates.

Fats have a crucial role in the absorption of fat-soluble vitamins, such as A, D, E, and K, in addition to providing energy. These vitamins are necessary for several physiological processes, including blood coagulation, bone health, and immunological function. Adequate consumption of healthy fats guarantees the assimilation of these essential elements, hence promoting general health and welfare.

Fats are essential parts of cell membranes as well. A particular kind of fat called phospholipids serves as the structural foundation for cell membranes, preserving their integrity and enabling a number of biological functions. Fats also have a structural role in the neurological system, where they are necessary for the development and operation of myelin, the sheath that protects nerve fibers and improves signal transmission.

Two particularly notable forms of polyunsaturated fats are omega-3 and omega-6 fatty acids, which are important for preserving cardiovascular health. The body is unable to generate these vital fatty acids, so eating is the only way to get them. Walnuts, flaxseeds, and fatty fish are good sources of omega-3 fatty acids, which have been linked to enhanced cognitive performance and a decreased risk of heart disease.

Although there are many health advantages to fats, it's important to pay attention to the kinds and quantities that are consumed. Overconsumption of trans and saturated fats has been linked to heart disease and other health problems.

Reduce your intake of trans fats, which are frequently included in partially hydrogenated oils used in processed foods and have a detrimental effect on heart health and cholesterol levels.

The idea of "good" and "bad" fats has changed over time, highlighting the significance of selecting healthy fats and limiting total fat consumption. Avocados and olive oil are rich sources of monounsaturated fats, which are known to have heart-protective qualities. Reduced rates of heart disease have been linked to a Mediterranean diet, which is defined by a higher intake of monounsaturated fats.

Individual dietary demands differ, so it may not be acceptable to take a one-size-fits-all approach to fat consumption. The ideal quantity and kind of fat in a person's diet depend on various factors, including age, sex, activity level, and general state of health. Seeking advice from a licensed dietician or healthcare expert can offer tailored recommendations based on specific needs.

An adequate diet that is both balanced and healthy must include fats. They help produce energy, facilitate the absorption of vital nutrients, and are crucial for preserving the composition and functionality of tissues and cells. Making educated decisions and choosing good fats while consuming fewer saturated and trans fats is crucial. It is imperative to adopt a well-rounded perspective on fat intake to enhance general health and wellness.

Chapter Two
Micronutrients Essentials

The hidden heroes of our diet are micronutrients, which are essential for cellular health maintenance. Although macronutrients like proteins, lipids, and carbs are given a lot of attention, micronutrients like vitamins and minerals are the unsung heroes of numerous physiological processes that are essential to human health. We examine the significance of micronutrients, their suppliers, and the effects of deficiency on human health in this investigation.

Recognizing Micronutrients

Micronutrients are composed of important components such as vitamins and minerals, which are necessary for many physiological activities but are required in relatively small amounts by the body. Organic substances and vitamins fall into two general categories: water-soluble (such as vitamin C and the B-complex) and fat-soluble (like vitamins A, D, E, and K). Conversely, minerals are inorganic elements that include but are not limited to, calcium, iron, zinc, and magnesium.

Vitamins: The Enzymes in Cells

In a variety of metabolic reactions, vitamins operate as catalysts, aiding in the creation of energy, the immune system, and tissue repair. For example, the manufacture of collagen depends on vitamin C, while energy metabolism is largely dependent on B-complex vitamins. Every vitamin has a distinct purpose, and deficiencies can result in a variety of illnesses, including beriberi and scurvy.

Minerals: The Foundation of Health

The fundamental components of many physiological structures are minerals. Zinc boosts the immune system, iron is necessary for blood oxygen delivery, and calcium is vital for healthy bones. The body's delicate homeostasis can be upset by an imbalance or lack of these minerals because they act in concert.

Micronutrient Sources:
A well-balanced diet is the main way to obtain micronutrients. A diet rich in fruits, vegetables, whole grains, dairy products, nuts, seeds, and lean meats helps supply necessary vitamins and

minerals. The micronutrients found in each food group are distinct, underscoring the value of diversity in the diet.

Deficiencies and Their Effects on Health:

Micronutrient deficits are common and can seriously harm one's health. Fatigue and weakness are the hallmarks of anemia, which can result from an iron deficit. Vitamin A deficiency can cause night blindness, whereas a vitamin D deficit is linked to bone problems such as rickets. Deficiencies are difficult to diagnose in the early stages because they frequently show subtle symptoms.

Immune Health and Micronutrients:

Micronutrients are essential for maintaining immunological function. White blood cell formation and function are improved by vitamin C, while immune response modulation is facilitated by vitamin D. A shortage of certain micronutrients can weaken the body's defenses against infections, making a person more vulnerable to disease.

Micronutrients All Through Life:
Micronutrients are critical for healthy living throughout the life cycle. Enough folic acid intake during pregnancy is essential for the fetus's neural tube to grow. Calcium and vitamin D are necessary for the growth and development of bones in children. Sustaining adequate amounts of specific micronutrients is crucial for sustaining cognitive function and averting age-related ailments as people age.

Micronutrients in Dietary Supplements:
Following special diets, such as vegan, vegetarian, or therapeutic diets, might make it difficult to consume enough

micronutrients. To guarantee that dietary requirements are satisfied, careful planning and, occasionally, supplementation are required. For example, vitamin B12 is mostly present in animal products, so vegans must take this into account when planning their diet.

Supplementation: A Contentious Method

Even though eating a balanced diet is the best way to get micronutrients, there are situations where supplements may be advised. The usage of supplements is still up for dispute, though, as taking too much of them can be hazardous. To prevent unforeseen repercussions, it is imperative to approach supplements cautiously and seek advice from medical professionals.

Obstacles to Accessing Micronutrients:

Even though micronutrients are important, not everyone has access to a varied, nutrient-rich diet. The availability and cost of foods high in micronutrients can be influenced by several factors, including geographic location, socioeconomic status, and cultural customs. It is imperative to address these differences to advance global health and well-being.

Taking Care of the Basis for Health: The unsung heroes that underpin our health are micronutrients. Their role is important, ranging from bolstering the immune system to supporting cellular activities. To fully benefit from micronutrients, one must make a deliberate effort to eat a varied and nutrient-dense diet and be aware of any potential deficits. A step toward promoting a healthier, more resilient global community is realizing the significance of micronutrients as we continue to explore the complexities of human nutrition.

4. Vitamins

Vitamins are necessary biological substances that are vital to many physiological processes in the human body. These micronutrients are essential for preserving well-being and averting certain illnesses. Even if they are not very necessary, their absence might have serious negative effects on health. It is essential to comprehend the many forms of vitamins, their sources, and their purposes if one is to promote general health.

Vitamins can be divided into two primary categories: fat-soluble and water-soluble. Vitamin C and the B-complex vitamins, which include thiamine (B1), riboflavin (B2), niacin (B3), pantothenic acid (B5), pyridoxine (B6), biotin (B7), folate (B9), and cobalamin (B12), are examples of water-soluble vitamins. These vitamins must be regularly ingested through a balanced diet because they dissolve in water and are not kept in the body for long.

Conversely, fat-soluble vitamins—such as A, D, E, and K—are absorbed in the digestive system together with fat and are subsequently deposited in the body's adipose cells. Extra fat-soluble vitamins, as opposed to water-soluble vitamins, can build up in the body and could cause toxicity. As a result, it's critical to keep things in balance and stick to daily allotment recommendations.

Every vitamin has a distinct purpose in the body. For example, vitamin A is necessary to keep the immune system, skin, and eyes healthy. Foods, including spinach, sweet potatoes, and carrots, contain it. Vitamin C is an antioxidant that is found in large amounts in citrus fruits, strawberries, and bell peppers. It also helps create collagen and strengthens the immune system.

Red blood cell production, brain processes, and energy metabolism are all impacted by the B-complex vitamins. B12 is mostly present in animal-based foods and is necessary for DNA synthesis and neuronal function. Folate, also known as vitamin B9, is found in leafy greens and legumes and is essential for healthy fetal development throughout pregnancy.

The body can produce vitamin D when exposed to sunlight, which makes it special. It is essential for the health of bones and the absorption of calcium. Vitamin D deficiency can cause diseases including osteoporosis and rickets. Vitamin E is an antioxidant present in nuts, seeds, and vegetable oils that aids in preventing cell damage. Last but not least, vitamin K, which is abundant in green leafy vegetables, is necessary for blood clotting and bone metabolism.

The main way to ensure that you are getting enough vitamins is to eat a balanced diet that is rich in different types of nutrient-dense foods. Supplements are useful for people who have certain deficiencies, but they shouldn't be used in place of a varied and well-rounded diet. Supplement overuse can result in imbalances and perhaps negative consequences.

The requirements for nutrients differ according to age, gender, health, and way of living. The needs of old people, children, pregnant women, and infants may vary. The majority of the time, a diet high in fruits, vegetables, whole grains, lean meats, dairy products, or dairy substitutes can supply all the vitamins required for optimum health.

Foods that have been fortified can help fill nutrient shortages in certain situations. For example, vitamin D fortification is frequently added to some cereals and milk products; this is especially advantageous for people who get little sun exposure. Nonetheless, to prevent consuming too much of a particular vitamin, it is crucial to pay attention to the total nutritional value of processed and fortified foods.

Deficits in certain vitamins can have detrimental effects on health. For instance, scurvy, which is characterized by weariness, swollen gums, and joint discomfort, can be brought on by a vitamin C deficiency. A lack of vitamin D is linked to weaker bones and a higher chance of fractures. Breathlessness, weakness, and exhaustion are symptoms of iron-deficiency anemia, a disorder linked to low vitamin B12.

On the other side, toxicity can result from consuming too much of several vitamins. For example, taking too much vitamin A can result in nausea, vertigo, and, in severe situations, even death. To prevent any injury, it is essential to know the maximum limits and suggested daily allowances for each vitamin.

Vitamins have an impact on emotional and cognitive health in addition to physical health. A few vitamins are necessary to keep the brain functioning normally, especially those belonging to the B-complex group. Folate, for example, is essential for the manufacture of neurotransmitters, and deficits have been associated with cognitive impairment.

Vitamins serve physiological purposes as well as aid in the prevention of chronic illnesses. Vitamins that are antioxidants, like C and E, aid in the body's defense against free radicals, which can otherwise cause cellular damage and the emergence of diseases like cancer and heart disease.

Vegetarians and vegans, for example, may need to be more mindful of their vitamin intake. It can be difficult to get vitamin B12 from plant-based sources because it is mostly present in animal products. To avoid deficiencies in such circumstances, fortified meals or supplements could be required.

Vitamins are essential for preserving good health and averting several illnesses. The basis for getting critical vitamins is a diet rich in a variety of well-balanced and nutrient-dense foods. Supplements are useful in some circumstances, but a varied and healthy diet should always come first. To fully reap the benefits of vitamins for general well-being, moderation in supplement use and awareness of individual nutritional needs are essential.

5. Minerals

Silent builders of our globe, minerals mold terrain, support life and conceal information that reveals Earth's geological past. These naturally occurring inorganic materials are what give rocks their structure and are essential to many industrial, commercial, and ecological operations. We learn about the wonders of mineral formation, their many applications, and their importance in both the natural and man-made worlds as we explore the complex world of minerals.

Creation and Variability

Millions of years of intricate interactions between various geological processes result in the formation of minerals. Crystallization, the process by which crystals harden from molten rock or precipitate from mineral-rich fluids, is one of the main ways that minerals are formed. Numerous different minerals with distinct crystalline structures and characteristics are produced as a result of this process.

With more than 5,000 identified species, the mineral world is immensely diverse, and new findings keep adding to our knowledge. These species are divided into several classes according to their crystal structure and chemical makeup. Minerals offer an astonishing diversity that captivates geologists, mineralogists, and enthusiasts alike. Silicates make up the majority of the Earth's crust, while other minerals include carbonates, sulfides, oxides, and more.

Geological Importance

Minerals offer priceless hints about the Earth's geological past. Scientists can learn more about the processes that molded the Earth's surface and the conditions under which these rocks formed by examining the minerals found in rocks. Geologists can determine the existence of extinct living forms, comprehend old climatic patterns, and even follow the evolution of landscapes through the use of mineralogical analysis. The study of index minerals, which serve as indicators of particular pressure and temperature conditions during metamorphic processes, is one well-known example. Over geological time scales, tectonic activities have sculpted mountain ranges and continents, and these minerals aid in the reconstruction of those events for geologists.

Economic Significance

In addition to their geological significance, minerals are essential to the world economy. Numerous minerals are vital raw materials used in a wide range of industries, from manufacturing and construction to technology and agriculture. While rare earth elements are essential components in electrical gadgets, metals like iron, copper, and aluminum are necessary for the construction of infrastructure.

For thousands of years, mining—the process of removing minerals from the crust of the earth—has been an essential human endeavor. The need for minerals increased as cultures developed, which resulted in the creation of complex mining operations all over the world. However, because mineral extraction can have negative ecological effects such as habitat destruction and water contamination, it also creates environmental issues.

Industrial Uses

Minerals are used in many different industries and are a common sight in our daily lives. The common mineral quartz is utilized in the creation of silicon chips and glass. Another mineral that is essential to the pharmaceutical and cosmetic industries is talc. Because of their special qualities, minerals are used in the production of anything from ceramics and abrasives to fertilizers and pigments.

A group of minerals known for their beauty and rarity are called gemstones, and they have artistic and cultural value.

Throughout history, jewels such as diamonds, rubies, sapphires, and emeralds have been used to embellish jewelry and have been symbolic of riches and prestige.

Environmental Difficulties

Although minerals are necessary for human advancement, the extraction and use of them present environmental problems. Mining operations are linked to deforestation, habitat degradation, and air and water pollution. Maintaining a balance between reducing the environmental impact of minerals and satisfying the world's expanding demand for them is still a challenge.

The creation of alternative materials, recycling programs, and sustainable mining techniques are essential steps in reducing the environmental impact of mineral extraction. A growing number of people are supporting responsible mining and consumption as environmental issues come to light.

 upcoming prospects
Exciting prospects lie ahead for the exploration and use of minerals. Technological developments like spectroscopy and remote sensing are completely changing how we find and examine mineral resources. These developments promote more sustainable practices in addition to increasing mining operations' efficiency.

 Furthermore, interest in mining beyond Earth has increased as a result of research into extraterrestrial entities like Mars and asteroids. There are scientific and commercial opportunities associated with the possible extraction of minerals from space resources, which could have an impact on future space exploration and settlement.

The unsung heroes that have shaped the past, present, and future of our world are minerals. Their creation, variety, economic value, geological relevance, and environmental difficulties weave a complicated web that is intricately linked to human society. We must work toward a peaceful cohabitation with the Earth as we continue to unravel the mysteries of minerals, understanding the fine line that separates progress from environmental care.

Chapter Three
Balancing a Busy Schedule and Nutrition

Maintaining a nutritious diet while juggling a hectic schedule is difficult but necessary for living a happy and healthy life. People frequently find themselves overwhelmed by the demands of work, family, and other commitments in today's fast-paced world, which makes it challenging to set priorities and maintain a well-balanced diet. For general well-being, it is imperative to comprehend the importance of nutrition and to adopt tactics that allow it to be easily incorporated into a busy lifestyle.

Realizing how important it is to provide our bodies with the correct nutrients is the first step in striking a balance between nutrition and a hectic schedule. To maintain overall energy levels, mental clarity, and physical health, proper nutrition is essential. People who don't eat well may get tired easily, be less productive, and be more vulnerable to certain health problems.

Meal planning is a useful tactic for maintaining a balanced diet in the face of a hectic schedule. Setting aside some time to organize your weekly menu will help guarantee that you are getting enough of these vital nutrients every day. This may include planning meals ahead of time, selecting easy-to-follow but wholesome recipes, and creating a shopping list to make grocery shopping more efficient. One way to resist the temptation to choose quick food options that are convenient but frequently unhealthy is to prepare your meals in advance.

Apart from making a meal plan, mindful eating is another technique that can help a lot with striking a balance between healthy food and a hectic schedule. Savoring every bite, paying attention to signals of hunger and fullness, and being mindfully present and attentive during meals are all components of mindful eating. This method not only improves eating experiences overall but also helps people digest food more effectively and make more thoughtful dietary choices.

Making sensible snack choices is another essential component of eating a balanced diet while managing a busy schedule. Nutrient-dense foods like fruits, vegetables, nuts, or yogurt can provide you with sustained energy throughout the day in place of sugary or processed snacks. Having wholesome snacks close at hand can help you make quick decisions when you're hungry.

Though sometimes disregarded, hydration is just as important to general health. A lack of water due to a busy schedule might affect one's ability to think, feel energized, and perform physically. Ensuring constant hydration can be achieved by incorporating water breaks into everyday routines, carrying a reusable water bottle, and setting reminders.

A healthy lifestyle requires making time for regular physical activity, even with a busy schedule. Exercise enhances mood and helps manage stress, in addition to promoting physical well-being. It can be simpler to stick to a regular exercise schedule if you mix in quick, intense workouts or select activities that suit your interests.

In terms of nutrition, variety is essential. A wide range of vital nutrients can be obtained by eating a variety of fruits, vegetables, whole grains, lean meats, and healthy fats. Adding variety to meals through the use of diverse cooking techniques and culinary explorations can keep meals from becoming boring and encourage a long-term commitment to a healthy diet.

When trying to strike a balance between a busy schedule and nutrition, it's critical to be flexible and realistic. There will be days when it's difficult to stick to a rigorous schedule due to time restrictions. Having a fallback plan, such as wholesome grab-and-go choices or easy-yet-nutritious meals, can be quite helpful in these situations.

Finding the right balance between a hectic schedule and a healthy diet takes deliberate work and dedication to putting one's health first. Meal planning, mindful eating, strategic snacking, staying hydrated, getting regular exercise, and consuming a variety of foods can all make a big difference in one's general state of well-being. People can manage their busy lives while preserving a solid foundation of health and vigor by realizing the significance of eating and implementing these habits.

6. Meal Planning Tips: A Guide to Effortless and Nutritious Eating

Meal planning has become a vital tool in the busyness of our everyday lives for maintaining a healthy lifestyle. It's more than just a fad; it's a sensible way to make sure our bodies get the nutrition they require without breaking the bank or taking too long. The nuances of meal planning will be covered in detail in this note, along with a thorough guide and helpful hints to make the process easier and more fun.

The process of arranging your meals with an emphasis on convenience, variety, and nutrition over a given time frame—typically a week—is known as meal planning. People can steer clear of the dangers of making snap decisions about their diet by taking the time to plan. Those with hectic schedules can particularly benefit from this practice, which will help them maintain a healthy diet without sacrificing time or energy.

Why Meal Planning Is Important for Nutritional Benefits: By allowing for a balanced distribution of nutrients, meal planning helps to ensure that your body gets the vital vitamins and minerals it requires. You can improve your general health and well-being by including a range of food categories.

 Time Efficiency: Making a weekly meal plan in advance helps you save a lot of time. Cooking is streamlined, less stressful, and more effective when you know what to cook and have ingredients on hand.

 Savings: Careful meal preparation might result in considerable financial savings. You may extend your shopping budget by purchasing products in bulk, taking advantage of bargains, and reducing food waste.

 Useful advice for meal planning
Make a Weekly Menu:
Plan your meals for the upcoming week first. Take into account your nutritional objectives, dietary choices, and timetable. Creating a menu gives you a detailed

plan for your food shopping and cooking tasks.

Accept batch cooking: make some recipes in larger quantities and freeze them in portion-controlled freezer bags for the week. This method guarantees that you always have handmade, healthy options on hand while also saving you time.

Incorporate a Range of Foods: To ensure that your meals cover a broad spectrum of nutrients, strive for diversity. Add a variety of fruits, vegetables, grains, and meats to your diet to make it vibrant and full of nutrients.

Keep It Simple: The secret to successful meal planning is simplicity, even though variety is vital. To prevent feeling overwhelmed, opt for recipes that call for simple ingredients and preparation techniques.

Prepare Ingredients Ahead of Time: Wash, cut, and divide ingredients into portions. The time and effort needed to cook meals over the week can be greatly decreased with this tiny investment in prep work.

Remain Aware of Portion Sizes: To avoid overindulging and reduce food waste, be aware of portion sizes. To determine the proper serving sizes, use measurement devices or visual cues.

Creatively Use Leftovers: To keep things interesting, repurpose leftovers into new dinners. For instance, use grilled chicken in a salad the next day or include roasted vegetables in a frittata.

Include theme evenings: Including theme evenings in food preparation would make it enjoyable. To reduce food waste, set aside a day for, say, vegetarian meals, an international cuisine day, or a "clean out the fridge" night.

Make a Comprehensive Grocery List: Following your meal planning, compile a detailed grocery list. Sort it according to dietary groups to make shopping easier and reduce the likelihood that you will forget anything important.

While planning is important, be adaptable and willing to make changes as needed. Having a flexible mentality enables you to modify your food plan in response to unforeseen events because life can be unpredictable.

Resources and tools for meal planning

Meal Planning Apps: Make use of meal planning applications that provide features such as grocery lists, recipe storage, and dietary data. These applications can help you plan more efficiently and generate ideas for new dishes.

Online Recipe Platforms: For a multitude of food ideas, check out online recipe platforms. Recipes are frequently categorized by dietary preferences on websites and apps, which makes it simpler to locate possibilities that support your objectives.

Cookbooks and periodicals: To obtain a tangible compilation of recipes, purchase a few trustworthy cookbooks or become a subscriber to culinary periodicals. Turning pages can sometimes inspire and stimulate creativity.

Participate in virtual forums and monitor social media profiles devoted to meal preparation and nutritious eating. Meet like-minded people to find new recipes, trade ideas, and share experiences.

A healthy, balanced diet can be achieved despite our busy lives with the help of meal planning. People may change the way they think about nutrition and make it a fun and sustainable part of their routine by implementing these suggestions and using the resources that are available to them. Whether you are a novice or an experienced meal planner, the secret is to discover a method that fits your needs and way of life so you can enjoy the rewards of conscious, wholesome eating.

7. Quick and Healthy Snack Ideas

Finding quick and healthy snack ideas is crucial for sustaining energy levels and general well-being in the fast-paced world of today. It's not necessary to associate snacking with consuming processed or empty-calorie items. You can have tasty and nutrient-dense snacks with a little preparation and imagination. This article will discuss a variety of quick and healthful snack ideas to suit a range of palates and dietary requirements.

1. Fresh fruit mix: A fresh fruit mix is one of the easiest yet most delicious snacks. Putting together a variety of in-season fruits offers a vibrant and nutrient-dense choice. Apples, berries, and slices of melon all have natural sugars that provide sweetness without the need for artificial sweeteners or preservatives. Combine it with a tiny bit of nut butter to get an additional source of protein and good fats.

2. Greek Yogurt Parfait: Yogurt provides a flexible foundation for a wholesome snack. Probiotics and high protein content help to maintain intestinal health. Layer Greek yogurt, granola, and fresh berries to make a yogurt parfait. This snack provides a balance of macronutrients to keep you energized throughout the day, in addition to satisfying your sweet craving.

3. Hummus and Veggie Sticks: A variety of fresh veggies go nicely with hummus, a tasty and protein-rich dip. Bell pepper strips, cucumber slices, and carrot sticks are also great options. Hummus is a filling and nutritious snack since it contains both protein and good fats.

4. Nut Mix: A personalized nut mix can be a quick and filling snack. Nuts that are high in heart-healthy fats include almonds, walnuts, and pistachios; cashews add a creamy texture. For natural sweetness, add a small amount of dried fruit, and for extra nutrition, add a variety of seeds. Because nuts are high in calories, pay attention to portion amounts.

5. Rice Cake with Avocado: Spread mashed avocado on top of a rice cake for a healthy, crispy snack. The fruit avocado is rich in nutrients and provides vitamins, minerals, and good fats. For added taste, add a splash of spicy sauce or a pinch of sea salt. This combination offers a pleasing texture blend and is easy to put together.

6. Hard-Boiled Eggs: Eggs that have been hard-boiled are an easy way to get protein and other necessary elements. To make a quick and portable snack, prepare a batch ahead of time and store it in the refrigerator. For extra taste, add a dash of sea salt or a small pinch of black pepper. Healthy fats and protein work together to ward off hunger.

7. Whole Grain Toast with Nut Butter: A traditional and wholesome snack choice is whole grain toast with nut butter. For extra fiber, use whole-grain bread and spread your preferred nut butter—almond, peanut, or tastemaker—

on it. A delicious blend of flavors is provided by the nut butter, while the fiber content encourages fullness.

8. Cottage Cheese with Pineapple: Cottage cheese is a dairy alternative that is high in protein and goes well with both sweet and savory toppings. Combine it with slices of fresh pineapple for a deliciously acidic and sweet snack. Cottage cheese's protein helps sustain a sensation of fullness while also aiding in muscle regeneration.

9. Veggie Wraps: Use lettuce leaves or whole-grain tortillas to quickly and healthily prepare a veggie wrap. Stuff them full of colorful veggies, hummus, and a lean protein source like tofu or grilled chicken. In addition to being filling, this snack provides a variety of vitamins, minerals, and antioxidants.

10. Dark Chocolate and Almonds: Dark chocolate and almonds are a tasty and reasonably decadent snack for people with sweet tooths. Almonds add crunch and good lipids, while dark chocolate has antioxidants. For the best results, choose dark chocolate with a higher cocoa percentage.

 Efficient and nutritious snacks are essential for sustaining energy levels and promoting general well-being. Without sacrificing flavor, these snack suggestions provide a good ratio of vitamins, minerals, and macronutrients. Try out several combinations to determine which ones work best for your dietary requirements and tastes. Snacking may be gratifying and healthy with a little imagination.

Chapter Four

Importance of Hydration

An essential component of preserving health and general well-being is staying hydrated. Since water makes up around 60% of the human body, staying hydrated is essential for several biological processes. We shall examine the significance of hydration in this note, including its effects on general vigor, mental clarity, and physical health.

Physical Condition:

The fact that hydration is essential for maintaining body functions is one of the main reasons. Every cell, tissue, and organ needs water to help with temperature regulation, joint lubrication, and nutrition transfer. Sufficient hydration guarantees proper organ function, fostering a robust cardiovascular system, streamlined digestion, and successful excretion of toxins via urine.

An enhanced immune system is also associated with proper hydration. Maintaining adequate hydration enhances the body's resistance against infections and diseases. White blood cells, which are vital for the immune response, are carried in lymph, a fluid that is produced with the assistance of water. Conversely, dehydration can weaken the immune system and make the body more vulnerable to illness.

Mental Process:
Sustaining mental clarity and cognitive function is largely dependent on adequate hydration. Because the brain is so

sensitive to variations in hydration, even a slight dehydration can hurt cognitive function. According to research, dehydration can cause mood swings, cognitive problems, and an increased sense of task difficulty.

The brain may momentarily shrink when dehydrated, impairing cognitive functions. Reaction time, memory, and focus can all be affected, which emphasizes how crucial it is to maintain proper hydration for mental health. Adequate hydration can improve the cognitive capacity of people working on tasks that call for creativity, concentration, or problem-solving.

Exercise Outcome:

Sustaining adequate hydration is essential for anyone who exercises, regardless of the intensity of their workouts or level of activity, to achieve peak performance. During physical effort, the body loses electrolytes and water through sweating. Fatigue, a drop in endurance, and cramping in the muscles are all consequences of dehydration.

After exercise, rehydration is crucial to replace lost fluids and stabilize electrolyte levels. The kind and intensity of their activity can determine the precise amount of hydration needed by athletes and fitness enthusiasts. Drinking enough water before, during, and after exercise promotes the body's healing process in addition to improving performance.

Controlling Weight:

The regulation of weight and total body composition are intimately related to hydration. Water is a great option for anyone trying to maintain or reduce their weight because it has no calories. Water consumption before meals may increase feelings of fullness and, hence, lower total calorie intake. Furthermore, enough hydration promotes the body's metabolic functions, which facilitate the effective utilization of nutrients for energy production.

Occasionally, the body may misinterpret thirst for hunger, resulting in the consumption of extra calories. Maintaining proper hydration can help people distinguish between hunger and thirst signals, which may support weight management objectives.

Skin Conditions:

The largest organ in the body, the skin, is greatly impacted by moisture levels. Dehydrated skin may seem flaky, dry, and more wrinkle-prone. Water is essential for preserving the suppleness and flexibility of the skin. Maintaining adequate moisture facilitates the removal of pollutants from the skin and aids in the skin's natural renewal processes.

To achieve glowing, younger-looking skin, staying properly hydrated is an easy yet crucial first step. Although skincare products are useful, they function best when used in conjunction with enough internal hydration.

Maintaining Hydration Balance:
Even though it's obvious how important it is to stay hydrated, finding a balance is crucial. Although it is uncommon, overhydration can cause hyponatremia, a disorder in which the body's electrolyte balance is upset. It is vital to monitor each person's specific hydration requirements, taking into account variables such as age, environment, level of physical activity, and health.

There is no way to emphasize how important being hydrated is. Water is a fundamental component of general well-being, supporting everything from cognitive function and physical functions to affecting exercise outcomes and skin health. One's health and vigor can be effectively and simply invested in by making frequent, adequate hydration a habit.

8. Water Intake Recommendations

Drinking enough water is essential for preserving general health and well-being. Since water makes up almost 60% of the human body, it is important for many physiological processes. Sustaining body functions, such as temperature regulation and nutrient delivery, depends on enough hydration. People should abide by specified guidelines on water intake to guarantee proper functioning.

Health professionals generally agree that each person should drink enough water each day to suit their individual needs. The Institute of Medicine (IOM) offers recommendations for the amount of water one should consume each day, accounting for variables like age, gender, degree of physical activity, and climate. These recommendations are an invaluable resource for ensuring appropriate hydration.

Age is one of the main factors taken into account when calculating water intake. For instance, an infant's water requirements differ from an adult's. Formula-fed newborns may need more water, particularly in warmer areas, but breastfed infants get most of their hydration from breast milk. Water requirements vary with age, and older people may be more susceptible to dehydration because of things like diminished thirst sense.

Another element affecting the amount of water needed is sex. Because of their differing bodily compositions, males typically require more water than women do. Men may have slightly higher water needs since they typically have a higher percentage of muscle mass than fat mass, and muscular tissue contains more water than fat tissue.

The degree of physical activity is a key factor in determining water consumption. People who work in physically demanding professions or exercise frequently need to drink extra water to replace the fluids they lose via perspiration. Staying hydrated is crucial when engaging in physical exercise, as dehydration can hinder performance and raise the risk of heat-related illnesses.

Water requirements are also greatly influenced by the environment and climate. Warm and muggy weather can cause increased fluid loss through sweating; therefore, drinking more water is necessary to stay well hydrated. People who live in colder areas, on the other hand, might not feel as thirsty, but they still need to watch how much water they drink.

The recommended daily intake of water, including all liquids and foods, is around 3.7 liters (125 ounces) for males and 2.7 liters (91 ounces) for females, according to the IOM. It's crucial to remember that every person has different needs. Some people may require more water because of things like pregnancy, certain drugs, or health issues.

Although these suggestions offer a useful starting point, it's important to listen to your body and recognize signs of thirst. People should not disregard their bodies' natural urge to drink more water—thirst is one of these signals. Furthermore, dietary factors—such as the use of alcoholic or caffeinated beverages—can affect one's level of hydration and necessitate modifying one's regular water intake.

Recommendations for water intake go beyond just how much water is drunk; water quality is also important. Maintaining general health and preventing waterborne illnesses require having access to clean, safe drinking water. People ought to be aware of the origin and condition of the water they use, choosing treated or purified water as needed.

 Following water intake guidelines is essential for preserving health. It's critical to recognize one's individual hydration requirements, regardless of age, gender, degree of physical activity, or environmental influences. Maintaining enough hydration and promoting general well-being requires striking a balance between consuming the recommended amount of water each day and paying attention to the body's natural cues. Promoting a healthy and hydrated lifestyle requires routinely evaluating and modifying water intake based on unique conditions.

9. Hydration and Energy Levels

A key component of sustaining ideal energy levels and general well-being is staying well-hydrated. It's important to acknowledge the significant influence that proper hydration has on our physical and emotional well-being in a society that frequently prioritizes hectic schedules and fast-paced lives. The complex relationship between energy levels and hydration is examined in this note, which highlights how crucial it is to maintain proper hydration for long-term vitality and optimal performance.

Water, which makes up a large percentage of the human body, is essential to many physiological functions. Water makes up over 60% of an adult's body weight, demonstrating how necessary it is. For optimal performance, all cells, tissues, and organs need to be adequately hydrated. Sweating is one of the main ways that water helps the body maintain a temperature, which is especially important when exercising.

Dehydration can have a significant effect on energy levels. Experiencing weariness and lethargic sensations can be a consequence of mild dehydration.

Hydration plays a crucial role in the delivery of nutrients and oxygen to cells, and dehydration can hinder this process and reduce the amount of energy produced. Studies have demonstrated that dehydration can have a deleterious impact on mood, focus, and cognitive function, underscoring the importance of preserving an appropriate fluid balance.
 Maintaining energy levels requires an understanding of the body's water requirements. Individual hydration needs are influenced by variables like age, gender, climate, and degree of physical activity. For example, athletes should pay special attention to the amount of fluids they consume because they lose water through sweat during strenuous exercise. On the other hand, elderly individuals could experience a decreased feeling of thirst; therefore, it's important for them to intentionally drink adequate water.

In addition to water, other drinks such as tea, coffee, and some fruits and vegetables can help you stay hydrated overall. But it's crucial to exercise caution when consuming alcoholic and caffeinated drinks, as they may have diuretic effects that raise the possibility of dehydration. The secret to keeping your hydration levels at their ideal level is to maintain a balance between different fluid sources.

Not only may dehydration cause physical symptoms, but it can also impair cognitive abilities. According to studies, even moderate dehydration might affect one's ability to focus, short-term memory, and make decisions. These cognitive impairments can have a major effect on day-to-day activities, productivity at work, and general quality of life. Therefore, staying properly hydrated is crucial for both physical and mental well-being.

Hydration affects energy levels at both individual and societal levels. For example, companies are realizing how important it is to encourage hydration in the workplace to improve worker well-being and Chapter Fovyproductivity. Easy access to water, frequent breaks, and promoting a hydration culture are becoming essential components of workplace wellness programs.

It is essential to inform people about the symptoms of dehydration and the value of taking preventative hydration measures. Although thirst is a direct indication that the body needs water, dehydration can sometimes prevent someone from experiencing thirst. For this reason, developing a habit of consistent fluid intake is crucial for long-term well-being, particularly when there are no thirst signals.

 Understanding personal needs and implementing them into every day routines is the first step toward developing appropriate hydration habits. Simple yet efficient tactics include picking foods that are high in water content, carrying a reusable water bottle, and setting reminders to drink water. Urine color can also be used as a rapid indicator of one's level of hydration; a pale yellow color indicates sufficient hydration, while a dark yellow or amber color indicates a need for additional fluids.

Sports drinks, which are frequently promoted as rehydration remedies, might be helpful in certain situations, such as prolonged periods of vigorous exercise lasting more than an hour. However, water continues to be the best option for regular hydration. It has no calories, is readily available, and is essential for sustaining general health and energy levels.

 There is no denying the connection between energy levels and hydration. Because the human body depends on water for vital processes and because dehydration hurts both physical and mental functioning, we must make being hydrated a priority in our everyday lives. Maintaining proper hydration is essential to realizing our full potential and leading vibrant, energized lives, whether at work, in the classroom, or during physical activity.

Chapter Five

Smart Food Choices for Energy

Sustaining adequate energy levels is essential for productivity, focus, and general well-being in the hectic pace of our everyday lives. Sugary snacks and beverages with a lot of caffeine may give you a brief energy boost, but the effects are usually fleeting and come with energy dips. Choosing foods wisely is crucial to maintaining energy levels all day. This essay examines the fundamentals of dietary selection that support long-lasting energy, emphasizing nutrient-dense foods and mindful eating practices.

Rich in Nutrients Foods

Complex carbs: A diet rich in complex carbs is essential for long-lasting energy. Whole grains, brown rice, quinoa, and sweet potatoes are examples of foods that release glucose gradually and provide you with a constant energy boost without the highs and lows that come with processed carbohydrates.

Foods High in Protein: Consuming foods high in protein during meals and snacks helps control blood sugar levels and increases feelings of fullness. Lean protein sources, including fish, poultry, tofu, and beans, can be great options for maintaining energy levels throughout the day.

Good Fats: Omega-3 fatty acids, which are present in walnuts, flaxseeds, and fatty fish, support brain health and may even improve cognitive performance. Healthy fats, such as those found in avocados and olive oil, can give you a slow-burning energy source.

Healthy snacks and meals

Regular Eating Schedule: Eating regularly helps control blood sugar levels and stave off energy slumps. Try to eat three balanced meals a day, including any necessary healthy snacks in between. Preventing extended intervals of fasting can aid in maintaining energy levels throughout the day.

Hydration: Being dehydrated might makeyou feel tired and less attentive. Maintaining proper hydration is essential for good body functioning. Good options for staying hydrated without added sugars are water, herbal teas, and infused water with fruits and herbs.

Mindful Portion Control: Avoid overindulging, which can cause energy collapses, by keeping an eye on portion sizes. A consistent supply of nutrients can be maintained with smaller, more balanced meals that don't tax the body's digestive system.

Meal Planning and Timing Strategy Breakfast: It's common to hear that breakfast is the most significant meal of the day. A healthy breakfast that consists of a mix of complex carbohydrates, healthy fats, and protein accelerates your metabolism and gives you long-lasting energy.

Mid-morning and Afternoon Snacks: Keeping energy levels stable between meals can be achieved by incorporating wholesome snacks. Choose protein-rich and carb-rich snacks, like Greek yogurt with fruit or almonds with whole-grain crackers.

Lunch: To avoid the mid-afternoon slump, eat a balanced meal. Consume a variety of veggies, lean meats, and nutritious grains to keep your energy levels up all day.

Supper: Choose a nutritious meal that consists of vegetables, lean protein, and complex carbs. Eating a lighter dinner can help to promote better sleep quality and avoid discomfort.

Conscious eating practices

Chew Your Food:

Eating slowly and fully promotes better digestion and enables the body to absorb nutrients more effectively. By eating mindfully, you can avoid overindulging and improve the absorption of nutrients.

Eat Less Processed Meals: Consuming a lot of processed meals can cause energy spikes and crashes because they are frequently high in refined sugars and harmful fats. A longer-lasting and more consistent energy release is guaranteed when whole, less processed foods are chosen.

Variety is essential.

A wide range of vital nutrients is ensured by consuming a variety of nutrient-dense foods. This variety gives the body the resources it needs for long-term energy and promotes general wellness.

A mix of nutrient-rich foods, balanced meals, and snacks, thoughtful eating practices, and meal scheduling is key to making wise food choices for long-lasting energy. You may maximize your energy, improve your ability to concentrate and advance your general well-being by implementing these ideas into your everyday routine. Recall that even little dietary adjustments can have a big impact on your long-term health and energy levels.

10.   High-Energy Foods

Eating foods high in energy is essential to maintaining an active and healthy lifestyle. It is impossible to overestimate the significance of providing our bodies with nutrient-dense foods in a society where people lead increasingly hectic lives. These foods give you the energy you need to keep up with your daily physical and mental tasks. In this note, we will discuss high-energy foods, their nutritional advantages, and how including them in our diets can improve our general health.

Foods high in energy provide a significant number of calories, mostly from fats, proteins, and carbs. The body needs these macronutrients to produce energy. Whereas lipids provide a more steady supply of energy, carbohydrates provide energy quickly and effectively. Proteins are essential for the growth and repair of muscles, as well as for general health and vitality.

The capacity of high-energy foods to deliver a rapid and long-lasting energy boost is one of their main advantages. Complex carbohydrate foods, such as whole grains, fruits, and vegetables, release energy gradually so that you have it all day long. Simple carbs are perfect for quick replenishment during strenuous physical activity since they can provide a quick energy boost. You can find them in foods like honey and fruits.

Despite being vilified in the past, fats are a necessary ingredient in diets high in energy. Good fats, such as those in nuts, avocados, and olive oil, help control blood sugar levels and promote fullness. They are also essential for the absorption of fat-soluble vitamins, including A, D, E, and K. Consuming a diet rich in fats in moderation promotes general metabolic health in addition to long-lasting energy.

Proteins, the building blocks of the body, are necessary for tissue upkeep and repair. Although they do not serve as the main energy source, a diet high in protein helps to maintain lean muscle mass and supports many physiological processes. Lean meats, dairy, legumes, and tofu are examples of foods high in protein that can be a vital component of a diet high in energy.

Including foods high in energy in our regular meals necessitates planning and balancing. Complex carbohydrates are found in whole grains like brown rice and quinoa, which offer a steady supply of energy. In addition to providing vital vitamins and minerals, fresh fruits and vegetables also provide a combination of simple and complex carbs that provide sustained energy.

Nuts and seeds are little energy-dense powerhouses that combine fiber, proteins, and healthy fats. A small serving of almonds or walnuts as a snack might provide you with a quick and wholesome energy boost. These foods also provide a variety of antioxidants and minerals that support general health.

A high-energy diet should consist primarily of lean proteins from plants like beans and lentils, fish, and chicken. These meals promote the health of muscles, help with the healing process following exercise, and increase feelings of fullness, which helps limit overindulgence in calories.

It's critical to consider the caliber of calories ingested. While foods high in energy are important, choosing foods high in nutrients guarantees that the body gets not just the energy it needs but also the vitamins and minerals required for optimal performance. Limiting processed and refined foods—which are frequently heavy in empty calories—can help prevent weight gain and have a detrimental effect on general health.

Another essential component of sustaining energy levels is staying hydrated. Water is essential for several physiological functions, including the metabolism of energy. The advantages of high-energy foods are enhanced when sufficient fluid consumption is maintained since it promotes healthy digestion, nutrient absorption, and general well-being.

Foods high in energy are essential to a balanced, active lifestyle. People can make educated dietary choices if they are aware of the significance of proteins, fats, and carbs. A varied, well-balanced diet rich in nutrient-dense foods gives you the energy you need for everyday tasks, improves your physical performance, and promotes general health and vitality. Making high-energy foods a priority as we manage the rigors of contemporary life is not just a decision but also essential to building a strong, resilient body and mind.

11. Foods to Avoid for Sustained Energy

Sustaining high levels of energy throughout the day is essential for both general well-being and maximum productivity. Although it's critical to include nutrient-dense meals in your diet, it's also critical to avoid items that cause weariness and energy collapse. This is a detailed list of foods to stay away from if you want long-lasting energy.

Highly Processed Foods: Refined sugars and harmful fats are common ingredients in processed foods, which can cause blood sugar levels to jump and fall quickly. To maintain steady energy, minimize your intake of sugary snacks, candies, and highly processed convenience foods.

Sugary Drinks: While energy drinks, soft drinks, and sugary juices could give you a temporary energy boost, the crash that follows can leave you feeling exhausted. For long-term hydration, choose natural fruit juices, herbal teas, or water with no added sugar.

White Bread and Refined Grains: White bread and pastries, which are manufactured with white flour, don't include the fiber that whole grains do. These may result in a sharp spike in blood sugar levels, followed by a decline. Select whole grains for sustained energy, such as brown rice, quinoa, and oats.

Overdosing on caffeine can cause jitters and energy dumps, but moderate caffeine consumption can improve attentiveness. Watch how much coffee, tea, and energy drinks you consume, and think about substituting them with water or herbal teas for healthier options.

High-Sugar Breakfast Cereals: A lot of commercial breakfast cereals are high in sugar, which causes blood sugar levels to drop after a brief energy boost. For longer-lasting energy, choose whole-grain, low-sugar cereals with extra protein.

Foods That Are Fried and Greasy: Foods that are fried and greasy, which are frequently heavy in bad fats, can be hard to digest and make you feel lethargic. For a lighter option, use cooking techniques like baking, grilling, or steaming.

Excessive alcohol use: Although some people may find moderate alcohol use acceptable, excessive alcohol use can cause dehydration, interfere with sleep cycles, and lower overall energy levels. Drink alcohol sparingly and keep yourself hydrated.

Artificial Sweeteners: Although artificial sweeteners, which are present in many diet products, don't contain calories, they can nevertheless increase cravings and interfere with the body's capacity to control blood sugar, which may cause swings in energy levels. Meats that have been processed, such as sausages, hot dogs, and deli meats, may have chemicals and preservatives that might exacerbate weariness and inflammation. Select lean, unprocessed protein sources such as beans, fish, and poultry.

Low-Calorie Diets: Excessive calorie restriction might result in low energy and nutrient shortages. Instead, to maintain sustained energy throughout the day, concentrate on eating a balanced diet that contains a variety of nutrient-dense meals.

Sustaining energy levels requires a diet high in whole, nutrient-dense foods and low in highly processed, sugary, and greasy foods. Maintaining proper hydration and portion control are also essential for meeting your body's energy requirements. Making thoughtful dietary decisions will improve your general health and guarantee that you have enough energy to get through the day.

Chapter Six

Exercise and Nutrition Synergy

Exercise and diet have a symbiotic relationship that is critical to pursuing a healthy lifestyle. Together, these two dynamic entities form the basis of well-being, impacting not just mental and emotional health but also physical health. It's clear from delving into the complex interactions between diet and exercise that their combined effect is much greater than the sum of their separate parts.

 Physical activity is a powerful inducer of physiological alterations in the body. The advantages are numerous, ranging from strengthened muscles to enhanced cardiovascular health. But to fully realize the benefits of these physical changes, careful consideration of nutrition is necessary. In addition to providing the body with fuel, proper nutrition also facilitates recuperation, therefore optimizing the benefits of exercise.

 Energy balance is one of this synergy's most important components. Regular physical activity raises the body's energy requirements. Sufficient nutrition supplies the required calories, macronutrients, and micronutrients, acting as the fuel for these tasks. Maintaining a healthy weight and promoting general well-being requires striking a balance between calorie intake and expenditure.

The three macronutrients—fats, proteins, and carbohydrates—have different functions in promoting both exercise and recuperation. The body prefers to use carbohydrates as its energy source, particularly while engaging in high-intensity activities. Proteins are critical for anyone doing strength training or endurance activities since they are necessary for muscle growth and repair. Good fats aid in the absorption of nutrients and add to energy reserves.

Optimizing the synergy between exercise and nutrition also requires careful consideration of the timing of nourishment. Meals before exercise give the body easily accessible energy, while nutrients after exercise are essential for restocking glycogen stores and speeding up muscle repair. Strategically organizing meals around training sessions boosts performance and generates better outcomes.

An essential component of this symbiotic interaction that cannot be ignored is hydration. Numerous physiological processes depend on water, and during physical activity, the body needs much more of it. Performance can be hampered, and the body's capacity to recuperate is compromised by dehydration. For this reason, maintaining appropriate amounts of hydration is crucial to optimizing the advantages of both diet and exercise.

Exercise and diet have a significant impact on mental health in addition to the physical realm. Frequent exercise is associated with better mood, lower levels of stress, and higher cognitive performance. These mental health benefits are enhanced by nutrition, which has an impact on neurotransmitters and brain function. Consuming a diet high in vitamins, antioxidants, and omega-3 fatty acids has a beneficial impact on brain function and emotional stability.

In terms of managing and preventing chronic diseases, exercise, and diet work in concert. A balanced diet and regular exercise can help reduce the symptoms of conditions including obesity, diabetes, and cardiovascular disease. Exercise increases insulin sensitivity, and healthy eating maintains cholesterol and blood pressure levels.

Exercise and nutrition regimens can be customized by individuals with specific fitness goals, such as weight loss, muscle gain, or sports performance, to get the best possible outcomes. Success depends on knowing one's calorie demands, nutritional needs, and the kind of exercise that will help achieve these objectives.

Seeking advice from a licensed dietician or healthcare expert can offer tailored recommendations based on personal goals and health circumstances.

The importance of this synergy increases as we negotiate the contemporary world of convenience foods and sedentary lives. Processed foods heavy in saturated fats and refined carbohydrates, together with extended periods of inactivity, are linked to several health problems. It will take a determined effort to incorporate regular exercise and a healthy diet into daily life to buck these trends.

The foundation of holistic health is the interaction between nutrition and activity. Their synergistic relationship affects mental and emotional health, illness prevention, and performance enhancement, in addition to the physical benefits. Accepting this mutually beneficial relationship gives people the ability to develop a way of life that nourishes their body and mind and promotes resilience and vigor for years to come.

12.   Pre-Workout Nutrition

Achieving fitness objectives and maximizing exercise performance depends heavily on a pre-workout diet. It's critical to comprehend the significance of consuming the right foods before working out, regardless of whether you're an athlete, a fitness fanatic, or someone trying to enhance your general health. This memo will explore the main points of pre-workout nutrition, such as its advantages, suggested nutritional intake, and useful advice to improve your workout.

Advantages of Nutrition Before Exercise:

Enhanced Energy: Your body can function at its peak when you fuel it with the correct nutrition before working out. Specifically, carbohydrates are a major energy source and can lessen weariness during physical activity.

Increased Endurance: By refueling muscles' glycogen stores before exercise, a healthy diet can improve endurance. This enables you to maintain your energy level throughout your exercise, allowing you to complete longer and more rigorous training sessions.

Increased mental alertness and attention: Some nutrients, like coffee, are well known for their capacity to increase mental alertness and attention. By incorporating these into your pre-workout routine, you can maintain mental clarity during your workout.

Improved Muscle Preservation: Eating protein before working out helps the body produce more muscle, which keeps the muscles from breaking down while exercising. For those who perform high-intensity workouts or resistance training, this is especially crucial.

Suggested Nutrients for Nutrition Before Exercise:

The body prefers to use carbohydrates as a source of energy. Before working out, consuming complex carbs such as whole grains, fruits, and veggies gives you consistent energy without shooting up your blood sugar.

Protein: Including protein in your pre-workout meal or snack helps to reduce muscle breakdown and promotes the synthesis of muscle protein. Choose protein sources that are simple to digest, including yogurt, lean meats, or whey protein.

Fats: Although they don't serve as the main energy source for intense exercise, fats do contribute to long-term energy production. Nuts, seeds, and avocados are good sources of healthy fats that can be included in your pre-workout diet.

 Hydration: For optimum performance, proper hydration is essential. Dehydration can cause cramping in the muscles, a loss of stamina, and problems with thinking. Before you begin your workout, make sure you are properly hydrated.

 Caffeine: It is commonly recognized that caffeine is a stimulant that can improve performance and attentiveness. It is frequently present in tea, coffee, and several pre-workout supplements. However, each person has a different tolerance for caffeine, so it's important to figure out how much is suitable for you.

Useful advice for nutrition before exercise:

The timing is crucial.

Try to have a well-balanced pre-workout meal or snack one to three hours before doing exercise. This enables the nutrients to be absorbed and digested by your body, giving you a steady supply of energy as you work out.

Customized Approach: When it comes to pre-workout nutrition, there is no one-size-fits-all strategy. When organizing your pre-workout meals, take into account your dietary needs, training regimen, and personal preferences.

Try Different Timing and Composition of Nutrients: See how your body reacts to various timings and compositions of nutrients. Try varying the amount of protein and carbs to see what affects your performance and energy levels the most.

Keep Yourself Hydrated: One sometimes-ignored component of pre-workout nutrition is hydration. Make sure you are well hydrated before beginning your workout, and if your training is longer than an hour, think about taking frequent breaks to sip water.

Think Carefully About Supplements: Although whole meals are the best source of nutrients, some supplements can enhance the nutrition you consume before working out. Before taking supplements, though, speak with a doctor or nutritionist to be sure they are appropriate for your needs and current state of health. A healthy diet before working out is essential to any fitness program. You can maximize your levels of energy, endurance, and overall performance by comprehending the advantages of appropriate feeding, including necessary nutrients, and adhering to helpful advice. Keep in mind that individual variations matter a lot; therefore, it's critical to customize your pre-workout diet to your unique requirements and tastes. Careful consideration of your pre-workout diet can have a significant impact on your overall health and performance, whether your objective is to reach peak sports performance or personal wellness.

13.   Post-Workout Nutrition

Any fitness plan must include post-workout nutrition since it is essential for maximizing muscle growth, recuperation, and overall performance. When people exercise, their bodies go through several physiological changes that necessitate adequate food replacement to promote recuperation and adaptation. In this note, we will discuss the essential elements of post-workout nutrition, as well as their significance and useful suggestions for optimizing the advantages of this crucial window.

The Significance of Nutrition After Exercise

Muscle Glycogen Resupply: Muscle glycogen reserves are depleted after vigorous exercise. After a workout, consuming carbohydrates replenishes glycogen, which facilitates quicker recovery and longer energy levels. Protein Synthesis: muscular protein synthesis is stimulated by post-exercise protein ingestion, whereas muscular protein breakdown is induced by resistance training. For the growth and healing of muscles, this is essential.

Reducing Muscle Soreness: Getting enough nutrition after an exercise might help reduce soreness in the muscles, lessen the effects of delayed-onset muscle soreness (DOMS), and enable people to train more frequently.

Hydration: Fluid loss occurs when exercising and perspiring. Rehydrating is an essential part of a healthy post-workout diet since it helps maintain fluid balance and guard against dehydration, which can impair performance and recuperation.

Important Post-Workout Nutrition Protein Ingredients:
To promote muscle protein synthesis, aim for 20–30 grams of premium protein. Lean meats, plant-based proteins (hemp, pea, and soy), and whey protein are some of the sources.

Glucose:

To replace glycogen levels, consume 0.5 to 0.7 grams of carbs per pound of body weight after a workout.

For long-lasting energy, choose complex carbs found in fruits, vegetables, and whole grains.

Fluids:

Rehydrate to replenish lost fluids and minerals using water or an electrolyte-containing sports drink.

Sufficient hydration promotes healthy cellular operation and the transfer of nutrients.

When:

It's generally accepted that the ideal window for post-workout nourishment is between 30 and 60 minutes following physical activity.

Eating nutrients during this time improves the body's ability to absorb and use them.

Useful Suggestions

Supplements versus Whole Foods:
For a well-rounded nutrient profile, natural foods should take precedence over supplements, even though they can be convenient.
Meals that are well-balanced and include protein, carbs, and fats support general health and healing.

Personalization:
Based on variables including age, weight, metabolism, and type of exercise, each person has different nutritional demands.
Adapt post-workout nutrition to individual preferences and goals.

Quality of Protein:
Select premium sources of protein to guarantee a full spectrum of amino acids.
Think about digestibility and allergies while selecting foods high in protein.

Strategies for Hydration:

Keep an eye on your fluid consumption throughout the day, not just after working out.

Beverages high in electrolytes are helpful, particularly after strenuous or extended exercise.

Proper Macronutrient Balance:

To satisfy your demands for general nutrition, keep your intake of fats, carbs, and protein in balance.

Specific objectives, like gaining muscle mass or decreasing body fat, can affect the distribution of macronutrients.

Frequently Held Myths and False Beliefs

Anabolic Window:

Although the timing of nutrients is crucial, the idea of a very small "anabolic window" has been contested.

Give your daily nutrient intake more importance than only the time you consume your meals after working out.

Overdosage of protein:

Increased muscle protein synthesis is not always the result of consuming an abnormally high protein intake all at once.
For best outcomes, spread out your protein intake equally throughout the day. Avoidance of Carbohydrates:
Particularly after exercise, carbohydrates are not bad for you. They are essential for the resupply of glycogen and the regeneration of energy.
Adjust your carbohydrate consumption based on your needs and objectives.
Nutrition after exercise is a dynamic and essential part of an all-encompassing fitness program. During this crucial time, careful consideration of nutritional intake can have a big impact on muscle growth, recovery, and overall athletic performance. People can use the advantages of post-workout nutrition to support their fitness objectives and foster

long-term well-being by recognizing the significance of important nutrients, customizing dietary methods, and busting common myths.

Conclusion

Now that you've finished the book, I hope you have a better understanding of nutrition and how it impacts your energy, performance, and overall health. Through this book, you have learned:

Your body needs three macronutrients: lipids, proteins, and carbs. You now know how to select the appropriate forms and dosages of every macronutrient based on your needs and preferences.

The vital micronutrients—minerals and vitamins—that your body needs. You now know how to support your body's numerous activities and functions by consuming enough of these nutrients through food and supplements.

How to manage your diet and hectic schedule. You now know some useful advice on how to organize your meals in advance, make nutritious snacks, and steer clear of typical mistakes that might negatively impact your nutrition.

The significance of water intake for your well-being and vitality. You now know how much water you should be drinking, how to check your state of hydration, and how your mood and energy are affected by hydration.

How to choose foods wisely to get energy. You now know how to manage your insulin and blood sugar levels, as well as which foods might increase or decrease your energy levels.

How to maximize the synergy between your diet and activity. You now know how to fuel your muscles and recover more quickly from workouts, how to avoid injuries and overtraining, and what to consume before and after.

Applying the knowledge and techniques in this book will help you become healthier, more energetic, and better nourished. You won't feel cheated or guilty, and you'll be able to appreciate your meals and life more. Recall that there is no one-size-fits-all approach to nutrition. You need to figure out what suits your body, your lifestyle, and yourself best.

After finishing this book, I strongly advise you to put what you've learned into practice. Build up your routines and habits gradually, starting with tiny, straightforward adjustments. Try new things and make adjustments as you go. And remember to acknowledge and appreciate your accomplishments.